The Vibrant Mediterranean Dinner Cooking Guide for Busy People

Get Ready to Amazingly Healthy and Fast Dinner Meals and Enjoy Your Diet

Ava Foster

© **Copyright 2021 - All rights reserved.**

The content contained within this book may not be reproduced, duplicated or transmitted without direct written permission from the author or the publisher.

Under no circumstances will any blame or legal responsibility be held against the publisher, or author, for any damages, reparation, or monetary loss due to the information contained within this book. Either directly or indirectly.

Legal Notice:

This book is copyright protected. This book is only for personal use. You cannot amend, distribute, sell, use, quote or paraphrase any part, or the content within this book, without the consent of the author or publisher.

Disclaimer Notice:

Please note the information contained within this document is for educational and entertainment purposes only. All effort has been executed to present accurate, up to date, and reliable, complete information. No warranties of any kind are declared or implied. Readers acknowledge that the author is not engaging in the rendering of legal, financial, medical or professional advice. The content within this book has been derived from various sources. Please consult a licensed professional before attempting any techniques outlined in this book.

By reading this document, the reader agrees that under no circumstances is the author responsible for any losses, direct or indirect, which are incurred as a result of the use of information contained within this document, including, but not limited to, — errors, omissions, or inaccuracies.

Table of contents

- CAJUN SEAFOOD PASTA 6
- SCRUMPTIOUS SALMON CAKES 9
- EASY TUNA PATTIES 11
- BROWN BUTTER PERCH 13
- FISH IN FOIL 15
- PEPPERONI EGGS 17
- EGG CUPCAKES 19
- HERBY JUICY CHICKEN FILLETS 21
- WILD RICE PILAF WITH BEANS 23
- ARROZ CON POLLO WITH A TWIST 25
- MACKEREL FILLETS WITH AUTHENTIC SKORDALIA SAUCE 27
- SICILIAN-STYLE BROWN RICE SALAD 29
- TRADITIONAL YELLOW RICE 32
- OLD-FASHIONED GREEK RIZOGALO 34
- ITALIAN-STYLE AROMATIC RISOTTO 36
- SAVORY MUSHROOM OATMEAL 38
- SPANISH REPOLLO GUISADO 40
- SPRING WAX BEANS WITH NEW POTATOES 42
- AJOBLANCO (COLD SPANISH ALMOND SOUP) 44
- SWEET SAUSAGE MARSALA 45
- FETA CHICKEN BURGERS 47
- BAKED SALMON WITH DILL 49
- HERB-CRUSTED HALIBUT 50
- MARINATED TUNA STEAK 51
- NIÇOISE-STYLE TUNA SALAD WITH OLIVES & WHITE BEANS 52
- TILAPIA WITH AVOCADO & RED ONION 55
- MIXED SPICE BURGERS 56
- DELICIOUS PORK & ORZO 58
- FLATBREAD SANDWICHES 59
- MEZZE PLATTER WITH TOASTED ZA'ATAR PITA BREAD 60
- MEDITERRANEAN WHOLE WHEAT PIZZA 62
- SPINACH & FETA PITA BAKE 63
- WATERMELON FETA & BALSAMIC PIZZA 64
- LENTIL, SHRIMP AND BEAN SALAD 65
- SPINACH AND EGG SCRAMBLE WITH RASPBERRIES 67
- MEDITERRANEAN LETTUCE WRAPS 68
- SHRIMP, AVOCADO AND FETA WRAP 70
- GREEK SALAD NACHOS 72

SIRLOIN WITH SWEET BELL PEPPERS	74
QUINOA AND SPINACH SALAD WITH FIGS AND BALSAMIC DRESSING	76
GREEK-STYLE TUNA SALAD IN PITA	78
DELICIOUS BROCCOLI TORTELLINI SALAD	80
TUNA AND CHEESE BAKE	82
PRESSURE POT POTATO SALAD	84
VEGGIE HUMMUS SANDWICH	86
SPICY POTATO SALAD	87
TOMATO AND HALLOUMI PLATTER	88
BEAN LETTUCE WRAPS	89
MARGHERITA MEDITERRANEAN MODEL	91
VERY VEGAN PATRAS PASTA	93
TANGY TILAPIA FISH FILLETS WITH CRUSTY COATING	95
FETA-FUSED MUSSELS MARMITE	97
SAUCED SHELLFISH IN WHITE WINE	99
MINTY MELON & FRUITY FETA WITH COOL CUCUMBER	101
LIMASSOLIAN LEMONY STEAMED SPEARS WITH CHEESE CHIPS	103
OVEN-GRILLED OYSTER MUSHROOM MEAL	104
GRILLED BURGERS WITH MUSHROOMS	106

Cajun Seafood Pasta

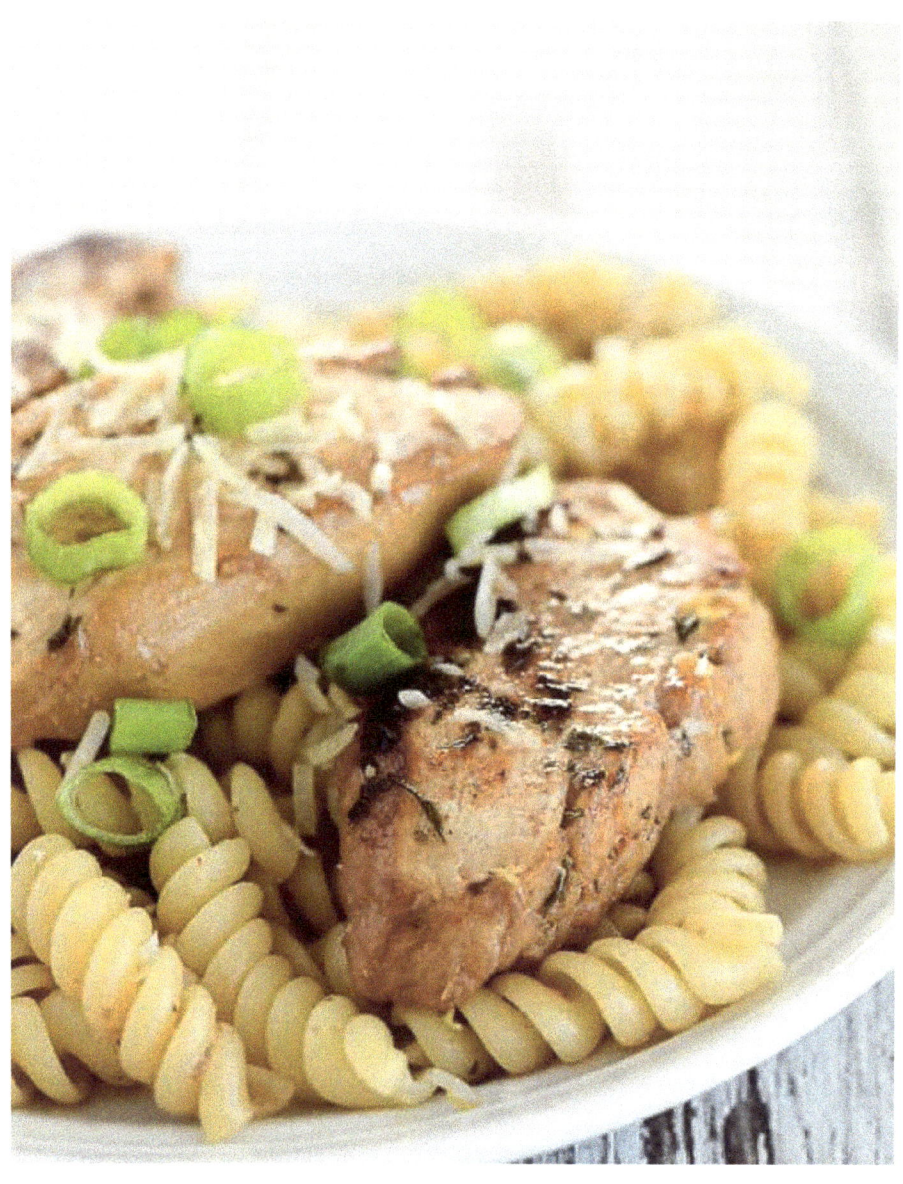

Difficulty Level: 2/5

Preparation time: 15 minutes

Cooking time: 8 minutes

Servings: 6

Ingredients:

2 cups thick whipped cream

1 tablespoon chopped fresh basil

1 tablespoon chopped fresh thyme

2 teaspoons salt

2 teaspoons ground black pepper

1 1/2 teaspoon ground red pepper flakes

1 teaspoon ground white pepper

1 cup chopped green onions

1 cup chopped parsley

1/2 shrimp, peeled

1/2 cup scallops

1/2 cup of grated Swiss cheese

1/2 cup grated Parmesan cheese

1 pound dry fettuccine pasta

Directions:

Cook the pasta in a large pot with boiling salted water until al dente.

Meanwhile, pour the cream into a large skillet. Cook over medium heat, constantly stirring until it boils. Reduce heat and add spices, salt, pepper, onions, and parsley. Let simmer for 7 to 8 minutes or until thick.

Stir seafood and cook until shrimp are no longer transparent. Stir in the cheese and mix well.

Drain the pasta. Serve the sauce over the noodles.

Nutrition: (Per Serving)

695 calories;

36.7 grams of fat;

62.2 g carbohydrates;

31.5 g of protein;

193 mg cholesterol;

1054 mg of sodium

Scrumptious Salmon Cakes

Difficulty Level: 2/5

Preparation time: 15 minutes

Cooking time: 10 minutes

Servings: 8

Ingredients

2 cans of salmon, drained and crumbled

3/4 cup Italian breadcrumbs

1/2 cup chopped fresh parsley

2 eggs, beaten

2 green onions, minced

2 teaspoons seafood herbs

1 1/2 teaspoon ground black pepper

1 1/2 teaspoons garlic powder

3 tablespoons Worcestershire sauce

2 tablespoons Dijon mustard

3 tablespoons grated Parmesan

2 tablespoons creamy vinaigrette

1 tablespoon olive oil

Directions:

Combine salmon, breadcrumbs, parsley, eggs, green onions, seafood herbs, black pepper, garlic powder, Worcestershire sauce, parmesan cheese, Dijon mustard, and creamy vinaigrette; divide and shape into eight patties.

Heat olive oil in a large frying pan over medium heat. Bake the salmon patties in portions until golden brown, 5 to 7 minutes per side. Repeat if necessary with more olive oil.

Nutrition: (Per Serving)

263 calories;

12.3 g fat;

10.8 g of carbohydrates;

27.8 g of protein;

95 mg cholesterol;

782 mg of sodium

Easy Tuna Patties

Difficulty Level: 2/5

Preparation time: 15 minutes

Cooking time: 10 minutes

Servings: 4

Ingredients

2 teaspoons lemon juice

3 tablespoons grated Parmesan

2 eggs

10 tablespoons Italian breadcrumbs

3 tuna cans, drained

3 tablespoons diced onion

1 pinch of ground black pepper

3 tablespoons vegetable oil

Directions:

Beat the eggs and lemon juice in a bowl. Stir in the Parmesan cheese and breadcrumbs to obtain a paste. Add tuna and onion until everything is well mixed. Season with black pepper. Form the tuna mixture into eight 1-inch-thick patties.

Heat the vegetable oil in a frying pan over medium heat; fry the patties until golden brown, about 5 minutes on each side.

Nutrition: (Per Serving)

325 calories;

15.5 grams of fat;

13.9 g of carbohydrates;

31.3 g of protein;

125 mg cholesterol;

409 mg of sodium.

Brown Butter Perch

Difficulty Level: 2/5

Preparation time: 15 minutes

Cooking time: 5 minutes

Servings: 4

Ingredients

1 cup flour

1 teaspoon salt

1/2 teaspoon finely ground black pepper

1/2 teaspoon cayenne pepper

8 oz fresh perch fillets

2 tablespoons butter

1 lemon cut in half

Directions:

In a bowl, beat flour, salt, black pepper, and cayenne pepper. Gently squeeze the perch fillets into the flour mixture to coat well and remove excess flour.

Heat the butter in a frying pan over medium heat until it is foamy and brown hazel. Place the fillets in portions in the pan and cook them light brown, about 2 minutes on each side. Place the cooked fillets on a plate, squeeze the lemon juice, and serve.

Nutrition: (Per Serving)

271 calories;

11.5 g of fat;

30.9 g of carbohydrates;

12.6 g of protein;

43 mg of cholesterol;

703 mg of sodium.

Fish in Foil

Difficulty Level: 2/5

Preparation time: 10 minutes

Cooking time: 15-20 minutes

Servings: 2

Ingredients

2 fillets of rainbow trout

1 tablespoon of olive oil

2 teaspoons of salt with garlic

1 teaspoon ground black pepper

1 fresh jalapeño pepper, sliced

1 lemon cut into slices

Directions:

Preheat the oven to 200 degrees C (400 degrees F). Rinse and dry the fish.

Rub the fillets with olive oil and season with garlic salt and black pepper. Lay each on a large sheet of aluminum foil. Garnish with jalapeño slices and squeeze the juice from the lemon onto the fish. Place the lemon slices on the fillets. Carefully seal all edges of the foil to form closed bags. Place the packages on a baking sheet.

Bake in the preheated oven for 15 to 20 minutes, depending on the size of the fish. The fish is cooked when it easily breaks with a fork.

Nutrition: (Per Serving)

213 calories;

10.9 g fat;

7.5 grams of carbohydrates;

24.3 g of protein;

67 mg of cholesterol;

1850 mg of sodium.

Pepperoni Eggs

Difficulty Level: 2/5

Preparation time: 10 minutes

Cooking time: 15 minutes

Servings: 2

Ingredients

1 cup of egg substitute

1 egg

3 green onions, minced

8 slices of pepperoni, diced

1/2 teaspoon of garlic powder

1 teaspoon melted butter

1/4 cup grated Romano cheese

1 pinch of salt and ground black pepper to taste

Directions:

Combine the egg substitute, egg, green onions, pepperoni slices, and garlic powder in a bowl.

Heat the butter in a non-stick frying pan over low heat. Add the egg mixture, cover the pan and cook until the eggs are set, 10 to 15 minutes. Sprinkle Romano cheese on eggs and season with salt and pepper.

Nutrition: (Per Serving)

266 calories;

16.2 g fat;

3.7 grams of carbohydrates;

25.3 g of protein;

124 mg of cholesterol;

586 mg of sodium

Egg Cupcakes

Difficulty Level: 2/5

Preparation time: 10 minutes

Cooking time: 20 minutes

Servings: 6

Ingredients

1 pack of bacon (12 ounces)

6 eggs

2 tablespoons of milk

1 c. Melted butter

1/4 teaspoon dried parsley

1/4 teaspoon salt

1/4 teaspoon ground black pepper

1/2 cup diced ham

1/4 cup grated mozzarella cheese

6 slices gouda

Directions:

Preheat the oven to 175 ° C (350 ° F).

Place the bacon in a large frying pan and cook over medium heat, occasionally turning until brown, about 5 minutes. Drain the bacon slices on kitchen paper.

Cover 6 cups of the non-stick muffin pan with slices of bacon.

Cut the remaining bacon slices and sprinkle the bottom of each cup.

In a large bowl, beat eggs, milk, butter, parsley, salt, and pepper. Stir in the ham and mozzarella cheese.

Pour the egg mixture into cups filled with bacon; garnish with Gouda cheese.

Bake in the preheated oven until Gouda cheese is melted and the eggs are tender for about 15 minutes.

Nutrition: (Per Serving)

310 calories;

22.9 g of fat;

2.1 g carbohydrates;

23.1 g of protein;

249 mg of cholesterol;

988 mg of sodium.

Herby Juicy Chicken Fillets

Difficulty Level: 2/5

Preparation time: 5 minutes

Cooking time: 20 minutes

Servings: 4

Ingredients

2 tablespoons olive oil

4 chicken fillets

1/4 cup red wine

3/4 cup chicken broth

Sea salt and freshly ground black pepper, to taste

1/2 teaspoon dried marjoram

1 teaspoon dried sage

1/2 teaspoon dried parsley flakes

1/2 teaspoon dried basil

Directions:

Press the "Sauté" button and adjust to the highest setting. Heat the oil and sear the chicken fillets for about 8 minutes, turning them over once or twice to ensure even cooking.

Pour in the red wine and scrape up the browned bits. Add the rest of the above ingredients.

Secure the lid. Choose the "Poultry" mode and cook for 5 minutes at High pressure. Once cooking is complete, use a natural pressure release; carefully remove the lid. Bon appétit!

Nutrition: (Per serving)

357 Calories;

18.4g Fat;

0.6g Carbs;

43.2g Protein;

0.3g Sugars;

0g Fiber

Wild Rice Pilaf with Beans

Difficulty Level: 2/5

Preparation time: 5 minutes

Cooking time: 30 minutes

Servings: 4

Ingredients

1 tablespoon olive oil

1/2 cup shallots, chopped

1/2 cup artichoke hearts, chopped

2 garlic cloves, minced

1 ½ cups wild rice

1/2 cup red kidney beans

3 cups vegetable broth

1 chili pepper, minced

1 teaspoon sage

1 teaspoon thyme

Sea salt and ground black pepper, to taste

2 ripe tomatoes, pureed

Directions

Press the "Sauté" button to preheat your Pressure Pot. Then, sauté the shallots, artichoke and garlic for 2 to 3 minutes.

Add the remaining ingredients to the inner pot of your Pressure Pot.

Secure the lid. Choose the "Manual" mode and cook for 20 minutes at High pressure. Once cooking is complete, use a quick pressure release; carefully remove the lid.

Ladle into individual bowls and serve warm. Bon appétit!

Nutrition: (Per serving)

384 Calories;

5.6g Fat;

67g Carbs;

19.4g Protein;

5.2g Sugars;

9.6g Fiber

Arroz con Pollo with a Twist

Difficulty Level: 2/5

Preparation time: 5 minutes

Cooking time: 15 minutes

Servings 5

Ingredients

2 tablespoons olive oil

1 Spanish onion, chopped

1 teaspoon garlic, minced

2 sweet peppers, diced

5 chicken drumsticks, boneless and chopped

2 cups water

1 cup cream of onion soup

2 Roma tomatoes, pureed

1 teaspoon Mojo Picante

1 teaspoon Spanish paprika

2 thyme sprigs, chopped

1 rosemary sprig, chopped

Sea salt and ground black pepper, to taste

1 ½ cups orzo, rinsed

Directions

Press the "Sauté" button to preheat your Pressure Pot; heat 1 tablespoon of olive oil until it just starts smoking. Sauté the Spanish onion, garlic, and sweet peppers until they are tender and fragrant; reserve.

Heat the remaining tablespoon of olive oil and adjust your Pressure Pot to the highest setting. Sear the chicken until golden-brown and crispy.

Add in the water, cream of onion soup, tomatoes, Mojo Picante, Spanish paprika, thyme, rosemary, salt, and black pepper.

Lastly, stir in the orzo and bring to a rolling boil.

Secure the lid. Choose the "Manual" mode and cook for 6 minutes at High pressure. Once cooking is complete, use a natural pressure release; carefully remove the lid.

Taste, adjust the seasonings and serve warm.

Nutrition: (Per serving)

435 Calories;

19.4g Fat;

37.6g Carbs;

28.7g Protein;

2.8g Sugars;

5.6g Fiber

Mackerel Fillets with Authentic Skordalia Sauce

Difficulty Level: 2/5

Preparation time: 5 minutes

Cooking time: 15 minutes

Servings 3

Ingredients

3 mackerel fillets

Sea salt and ground black pepper, to taste

1/2 teaspoon paprika

1 lemon, sliced

Skordalia Sauce:

4 cloves garlic

1/2 teaspoon sea salt

2 mashed potatoes

4 tablespoons olive oil

2 tablespoons wine vinegar

Directions

Place 1/2 lemon and 1 cup of water in the inner pot. Place the rack on top. Arrange the mackerel fillets on the rack.

Sprinkle salt, black pepper, and paprika over the mackerel fillets.

Secure the lid. Choose the "Manual" mode and cook for 4 minutes at High pressure. Once cooking is complete, use a quick pressure release; carefully remove the lid.

Meanwhile, make the sauce by blending all of the ingredients in your food processor.

Garnish the mackerel fillets with the remaining lemon slices and serve with the Skordalia sauce on the side. Enjoy!

Nutrition: (Per serving)

517 Calories;

33.6g Fat;

28g Carbohydrates;

24.3g Protein;

2.4g Sugars;

3.6g Fiber

Sicilian-Style Brown Rice Salad

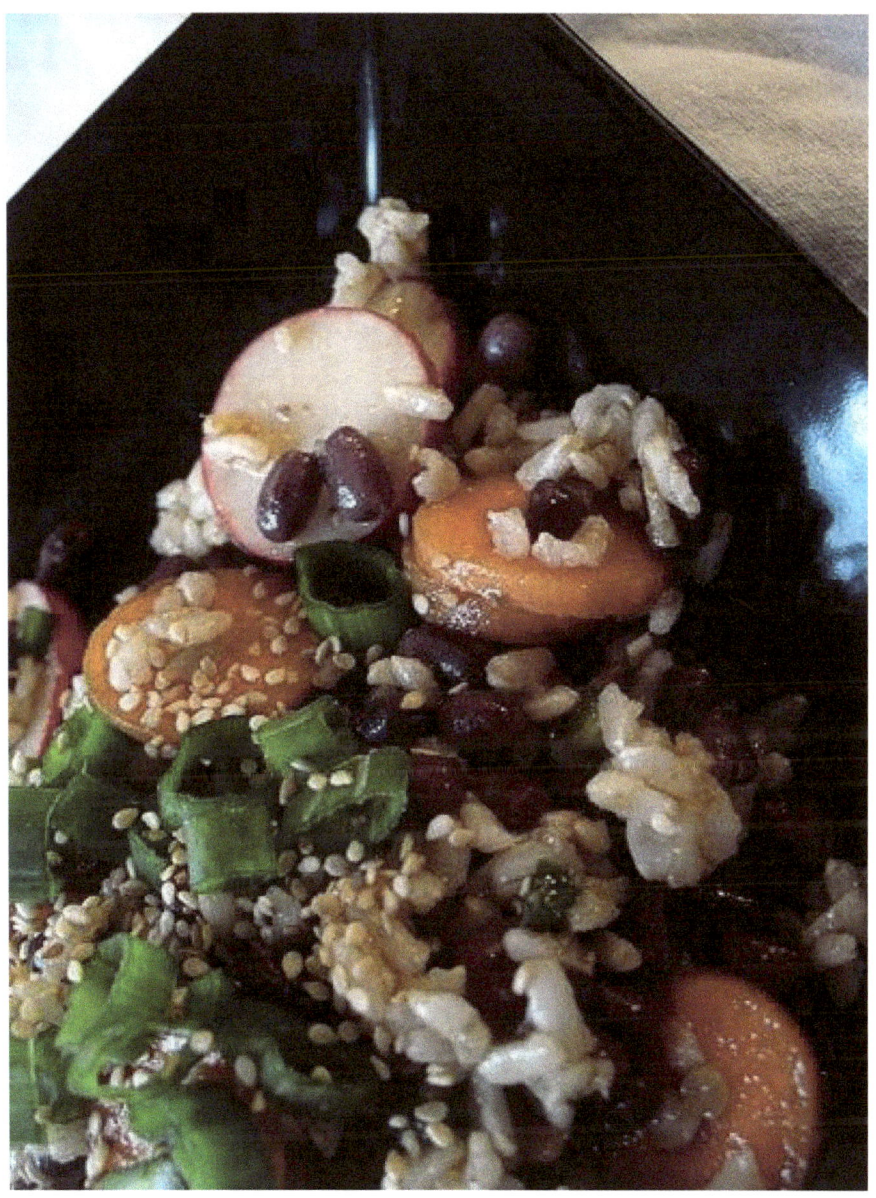

Difficulty Level: 2/5

Preparation time: 5 minutes

Cooking time: 20 minutes

Servings 4

Ingredients

2 cups vegetable broth

1 ½ cups brown rice, rinsed

1/3 pound asparagus spears

1 purple onion, sliced

1/2 cup sun-dried tomatoes in oil, drained and chopped

1/4 cup ripe olives, pitted and halved

Vinaigrette:

1/2 teaspoon fresh dill, minced

1/2 teaspoon fresh rosemary, minced

Sea salt and ground black pepper, to taste

1 tablespoon yellow mustard

4 tablespoons olive oil

1/2 lemon, zested and juiced

1 teaspoon garlic, minced

Directions

Place the vegetable broth and brown rice in the inner pot of your Pressure Pot.

Secure the lid. Choose the "Manual" mode and cook for 13 minutes at High pressure. Once cooking is complete, use a natural pressure release; carefully remove the lid.

Add the asparagus spears to the inner pot and seal the lid again. Choose the "Manual" mode and cook for 2 minutes at High pressure.

Once cooking is complete, use a quick pressure release; carefully remove the lid.

Transfer the cooked rice and asparagus to a serving bowl; add the purple onion, sun-dried tomatoes, and olives to the bowl and toss to combine.

Mix all ingredients for the vinaigrette; dress your salad and enjoy!

Nutrition: (Per serving)

457 Calories;

19.3g Fat;

62.3g Carbs;

10.4g Protein;

2.6g Sugars;

5.2g Fiber

Traditional Yellow Rice

Difficulty Level: 2/5

Preparation time: 5 minutes

Cooking time: 20 minutes

Servings 4

Ingredients

Ground black pepper, to taste

1/2 teaspoon cayenne pepper

1/2 teaspoon celery seeds

1/2 teaspoon turmeric powder

1 bay laurel

1 cup vegetable broth

1 cup jasmine rice, rinsed

2 tablespoons ghee, melted

Directions

Add all of the above ingredients, except for the ghee, to the inner pot of your Pressure Pot.

Secure the lid. Choose the "Manual" mode and cook for 9 minutes at High pressure. Once cooking is complete, use a natural pressure release for 10 minutes; carefully remove the lid.

Drizzle the melted ghee over each serving and enjoy!

Nutrition: (Per serving)

158 Calories;

12.3g Fat;

15.7g Carbs;

0.4g Protein;

2.6g Sugars;

6.5g Fiber

Old-Fashioned Greek Rizogalo

Difficulty Level: 2/5

Preparation time: 5 minutes

Cooking time: 20 minutes

Servings 4

Ingredients

1/4 teaspoon ground cardamom

1/8 teaspoon freshly grated nutmeg

1/2 teaspoon ground allspice berries

1/2 teaspoon ground cinnamon

1 teaspoon orange zest

1 cup white long-grain rice

1 ½ cups almond milk

2 tablespoons honey

4 tablespoons black currants

4 tablespoons almonds, slivered

Directions

Place the ground cardamom, nutmeg, allspice, cinnamon, orange zest, white rice, and almond milk in the inner pot of your Pressure Pot.

Secure the lid. Choose the "Rice" mode and cook for 12 minutes at High pressure. Once cooking is complete, use a natural pressure release for 10 minutes; carefully remove the lid.

Spoon your rizogalo into individual bowls. Garnish with honey, black currants and almonds and serve warm.

Nutrition: (Per serving)

260 Calories;

2.2g Fat;

56.1g Carbs;

4.4g Protein;

17.2g Sugars;

1.4g Fiber

Italian-Style Aromatic Risotto

Difficulty Level: 2/5

Preparation time: 5 minutes

Cooking time: 20 minutes

Servings 5

Ingredients

1 ½ cups Arborio rice

1/4 teaspoon ground bay laurel

1/4 teaspoon mustard seeds

1/2 teaspoon oregano

1/2 teaspoon basil

1/2 teaspoon thyme

2 cups roasted vegetable broth

1 cup Parmigiano-Reggiano cheese, preferably freshly grated

Directions

Place all ingredients, except for the Parmigiano-Reggiano cheese, in the inner pot of your Pressure Pot.

Secure the lid. Choose the "Rice" mode and cook for 12 minutes at High pressure. Once cooking is complete, use a natural pressure release for 10 minutes; carefully remove the lid.

Ladle into serving bowls, garnish with cheese and serve immediately. Bon appétit!

Nutrition: (Per serving)

295 Calories;

8.1g Fat;

44.1g Carbs;

10.8g Protein;

1.1g Sugars;

2g Fiber

Savory Mushroom Oatmeal

Difficulty Level: 2/5

Preparation time: 5 minutes

Cooking time: 15 minutes

Servings 4

Ingredients

1 tablespoon olive oil

2 cups button mushrooms, chopped

1 garlic clove, minced

2 scallion stalks, chopped

1 ½ cups rolled oats

2 cups water

1 ½ cups cream of mushroom soup

1/2 teaspoon turmeric powder

1/2 teaspoon cumin

1/4 teaspoon fennel seeds

1/4 teaspoon mustard seeds

Coarse sea salt and ground black pepper, to taste

Directions

Press the "Sauté" button to preheat your Pressure Pot. Heat the oil until sizzling. Now, sauté the mushrooms, garlic, and scallions until they have softened.

Add in the remaining ingredients; stir to combine.

Secure the lid. Choose the "Manual" mode and cook for 5 minutes at High pressure. Once cooking is complete, use a natural pressure release for 10 minutes; carefully remove the lid.

Spoon into individual bowls and serve warm. Bon appétit!

Nutrition: (Per serving)

360 Calories;

12.7g Fat;

49g Carbs;

14.3g Protein;

1.3g Sugars;

7.4g Fiber

Spanish Repollo Guisado

Difficulty Level: 2/5

Preparation time: 5 minutes

Cooking time: 10 minutes

Servings 5

Ingredients

2 tablespoons olive oil

1 large-sized Spanish onion, chopped

2 garlic cloves, minced

1/2 teaspoon cumin seeds

1 cup tomato sauce

1 cup water

2 tablespoons vegetable bouillon granules

1 tablespoon white wine vinegar

1/4 teaspoon ground bay leaf

1 teaspoon Spanish paprika

1/4 teaspoon ground black pepper, to taste

Sea salt, to taste

2 pounds purple cabbage, slice into wedges

Directions

Press the "Sauté" button to preheat your Pressure Pot; heat the olive oil. Once hot, sauté the Spanish onion until it is tender and translucent.

Add in the garlic and cumin seeds; continue to sauté an additional minute, stirring frequently. Stir the remaining ingredients, minus the vinegar, into the inner pot of your Pressure Pot.

Secure the lid. Choose the "Manual" mode and cook for 5 minutes at High pressure. Once cooking is complete, use a quick pressure release; carefully remove the lid.

Nutrition: (Per serving)

191 Calories;

6.4g Fat;

29.8g Carbohydrates;

5.1g Protein;

14.4g Sugars;

7.8g Fiber

Spring Wax Beans with New Potatoes

Difficulty Level: 2/5

Preparation time: 5 minutes

Cooking time: 20 minutes

Servings 3

Ingredients

1 tablespoon olive oil

2 scallion stalks, chopped

5 new potatoes, scrubbed and halved

1 sweet pepper, seeded and sliced

2 green garlic stalks, chopped

1/2 cup tomato sauce

2 tablespoons tomato paste

1/2 teaspoon brown sugar

1/2 cup roasted vegetable broth

1 pound wax beans, trimmed

Sea salt and ground black pepper, to taste

Directions

Press the "Sauté" button to preheat your Pressure Pot; heat the olive oil until sizzling. Now, sauté the scallions and new potatoes until just tender and fragrant.

Stir in the sweet pepper and green garlic and continue to sauté an additional 30 seconds.

Add in the tomato sauce, tomato paste, brown sugar, vegetable broth, and wax beans. Season with salt and black pepper.

Secure the lid. Choose the "Manual" mode and cook for 3 minutes at High pressure. Once cooking is complete, use a natural pressure release for 10 minutes; carefully remove the lid.

Taste, adjust seasonings and serve. Bon appétit!

Nutrition: (Per serving)

399 Calories;

5.6g Fat;

80g Carbs;

11.4g Protein;

15.8g Sugars;

13.5g Fiber

Ajoblanco (Cold Spanish Almond Soup)

Difficulty Level: 2/5

Preparation & Cooking Time: 25 minutes

Servings: 4

Ingredients:

Blanched almonds (1 lb.)

Red wine vinegar (3 tbsp.)

Olive oil (6 tbsp.)

Ice-cold water (3 tbsp.)

Garlic (1 clove)

Salt (as desired)

Green grapes (.25 cup)

Directions:

Mince the garlic and peel the grapes.

Combine the oil, almonds, vinegar, water, salt, and garlic in a blender until it's creamy, adding water as needed to keep it thick, but pourable.

Wait for about 15 minutes and chill the delicious soup before garnishing with the grapes.

Nutrition:

Calories: 853

Protein: 25 grams

Fat: 77.8 grams

Sweet Sausage Marsala

Difficulty Level: 2/5

Preparation & Cooking Time: 25-30 minutes

Servings: 6

Ingredients:

Italian sausage links (1 lb.)

Green and red bell pepper (1 medium of each color)

Tomatoes (14.5 oz. can)

Large onion (half of 1)

Garlic (.5 tsp.)

Dried oregano (.125 tsp.)

Black pepper (.125 tsp.)

Marsala wine (1 tbsp.)

Water (.33 cup)

Uncooked bow-tie pasta (16 oz.)

Directions:

Slice the onion and green peppers. Dice the garlic.

Prepare a large soup pot or other pot of boiling water - about half full. Toss in the pasta and simmer for about eight to ten minutes.

Meanwhile, add the sausage to a medium skillet and pour in the water. Set the temperature using the med-high heat temperature. Put a top on the pot and simmer for eight minutes.

When the pasta is done, drain it into a colander and set it to the side for now.

Drain the sausage and return to the skillet. Stir in the wine, garlic, onion, and peppers. Simmer it for about five minutes using the med-high temperature setting or until done.

Empty in the tomatoes, oregano, and black pepper.

Add the pasta and continue stirring. Serve and enjoy it anytime.

Nutrition:

Calories: 509

Protein: 21.9 grams

Fat: 16.1 grams

Feta Chicken Burgers

Difficulty Level: 2/5

Preparation & Cooking Time: 30 minutes

Servings: 6

Ingredients:

Reduced-fat mayonnaise (.25 cup)

Finely chopped cucumber (.25 cup)

Black pepper (.25 tsp.)

Garlic powder (1 tsp.)

Chopped roasted sweet red pepper (.5 cup)

Greek seasoning (.5 tsp.)

Lean ground chicken (1.5 lb.)

Crumbled feta cheese (1 cup)

Whole wheat burger buns (6 toasted)

Directions:

Heat the broiler to the oven ahead of time. Combine the mayo and cucumber. Set aside.

Whisk each of the seasonings and the red pepper for the burgers. Work in the chicken and the cheese. Shape the mixture into six ½-inch thick patties.

Broil the burgers approximately four inches from the heat source. It should take about three to four minutes per side until the thermometer reaches 165° Fahrenheit.

Serve on the buns with the cucumber sauce. Top it off with tomato and lettuce if desired and serve.

Nutrition:

Calories: 356

Protein: 31 grams

Fat: 14 grams

Baked Salmon with Dill

Difficulty Level: 2/5

Preparation & Cooking Time: 15 minutes

Servings: 4

Ingredients:

Salmon fillets (4- 6 oz. portions - 1-inch thickness)

Kosher salt (.5 tsp.)

Finely chopped fresh dill (1.5 tbsp.)

Black pepper (.125 tsp.)

Lemon wedges (4)

Directions:

Warm the oven in advance to reach 350° Fahrenheit.

Lightly grease a baking sheet with a misting of cooking oil spray and add the fish. Lightly spritz the fish with the spray along with a shake of salt, pepper, and dill.

Bake it until the fish is easily flaked (10 min.).

Serve with lemon wedges.

Nutrition:

Calories: 251

Protein: 28 grams

Fat: 16 grams

Herb-Crusted Halibut

Difficulty Level: 2/5

Preparation & Cooking Time: 25 minutes

Servings: 4

Ingredients:

Fresh parsley (.33 cup)

Fresh dill (.25 cup)

Fresh chives (.25 cup)

Lemon zest (1 tsp.)

Panko breadcrumbs (.75 cup)

Olive oil (1 tbsp.)

Freshly cracked black pepper (.25 tsp.)

Sea salt (1 tsp.)

Halibut fillets (4 - 6 oz.)

Directions:

Chop the fresh dill, chives, and parsley. Prepare a baking tray using a sheet of foil. Set the oven to reach 400° Fahrenheit.

Combine the salt, pepper, lemon zest, olive oil, chives, dill, parsley, and the breadcrumbs in a mixing bowl.

Rinse the halibut thoroughly. Use paper towels to dry it before baking.

Arrange the fish on the baking sheet. Spoon the crumbs over the fish and press it into each of the fillets.

Bake it until the top is browned and easily flaked or about 10 to 15 minutes.

Nutrition:

Calories: 273

Protein: 38 grams

Fat: 7 grams

Marinated Tuna Steak

Difficulty Level: 2/5

Preparation & Cooking Time: 15-20 minutes

Serving: 4

Ingredients:

Olive oil (2 tbsp.)

Orange juice (.25 cup)

Soy sauce (.25 cup)

Lemon juice (1 tbsp.)

Fresh parsley (2 tbsp.)

Garlic clove (1)

Ground black pepper (.5 tsp.)

Fresh oregano (.5 tsp.)

Tuna steaks (4 - 4 oz. steaks)

Directions:

Mince the garlic and chop the oregano and parsley.

In a glass container, mix the pepper, oregano, garlic, parsley, lemon juice, soy sauce, olive oil, and orange juice.

Warm the grill using the high heat setting. Grease the grate with oil.

Add to tuna steaks and cook for five to six minutes. Turn and baste with the marinated sauce.

Cook another five minutes or until it's the way you like it. Discard the remaining marinade.

Nutrition:

Calories: 200

Protein: 27.4 grams

Fat: 7.9 grams

Niçoise-Style Tuna Salad With Olives & White Beans

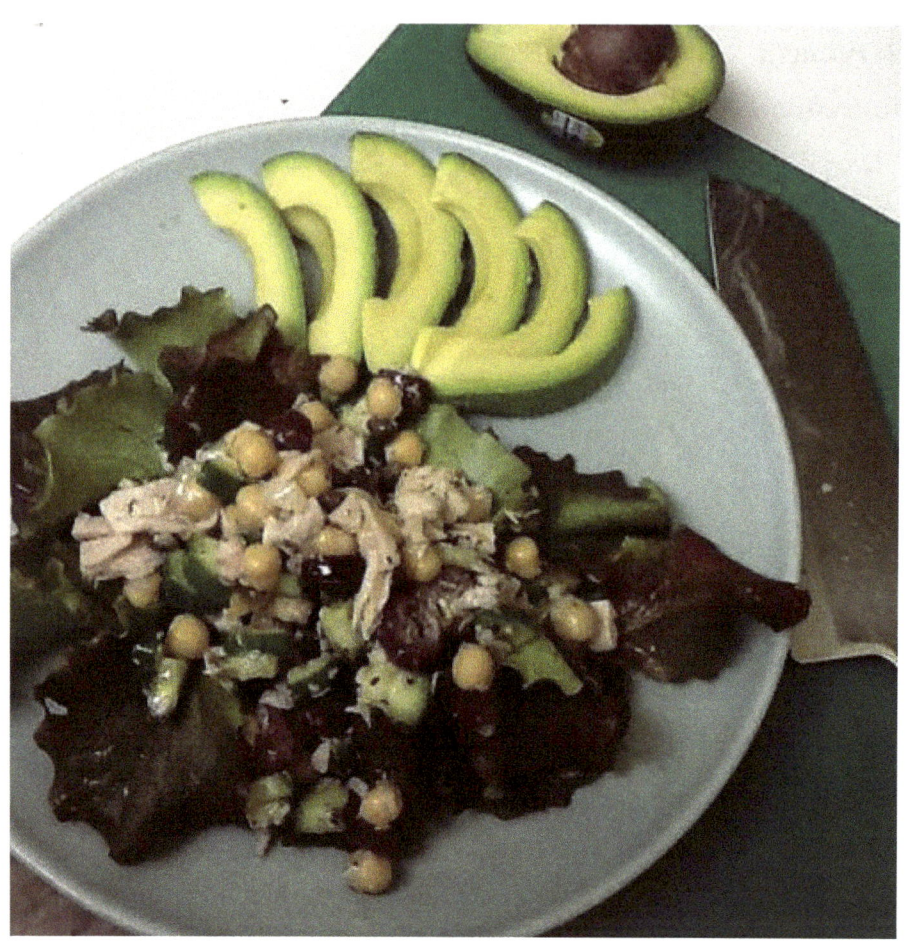

Difficulty Level: 2/5

Preparation & Cooking Time: 20-30 minutes

Servings: 4

Ingredients Needed:

Green beans (.75 lb.)

Solid white albacore tuna (12 oz. can)

Great Northern beans (16 oz. can)

Sliced black olives (2.25 oz.)

Thinly sliced medium red onion (¼ of 1)

Hard-cooked eggs (4 large)

Dried oregano (1 tsp.)

Olive oil (6 tbsp.)

Black pepper and salt (as desired)

Finely grated lemon zest (.5 tsp.)

Water (.33 cup)

Lemon juice (3 tbsp.)

Directions:

Drain the can of tuna, Great Northern beans, and black olives. Trim and snap the green beans into halves. Thinly slice the red onion. Cook and peel the eggs until hard-boiled.

Pour the water and salt into a skillet and add the beans. Place a top on the pot and switch the temperature setting to high. Wait for it to boil.

Once the beans are cooking, set a timer for five minutes. Immediately, drain and add the beans to a cookie sheet with a raised edge on paper towels to cool.

Combine the onion, olives, white beans, and drained tuna. Mix them with the zest, lemon juice, oil, and oregano.

Dump the mixture over the salad and gently toss.

Adjust the seasonings to your liking. Portion the tuna-bean salad with the green beans and eggs to serve.

Nutrition:

Calories: 548

Protein: 36.3 grams

Fat: 30.3 grams

Tilapia with Avocado & Red Onion

Difficulty Level: 2/5

Preparation & Cooking Time: 15 minutes

Servings: 4

Ingredients:

Olive oil (1 tbsp.)

Sea salt (.25 tsp.)

Fresh orange juice (1 tbsp.)

Tilapia fillets (four 4 oz. - more rectangular than square)

Red onion (.25 cup)

Sliced avocado (1)

Also Needed: 9-inch pie plate

Directions:

Combine the salt, juice, and oil to add into the pie dish. Work with one fillet at a time. Place it in the dish and turn to coat all sides.

Arrange the fillets in a wagon wheel-shaped formation. (Each of the fillets should be in the center of the dish with the other end draped over the edge.)

Place a tablespoon of the onion on top of each of the fillets and fold the end into the center. Cover the dish with plastic wrap, leaving one corner open to vent the steam.

Place in the microwave using the high heat setting for three minutes. It's done when the center can be easily flaked.

Top the fillets off with avocado and serve.

Nutrition:

Calories: 200

Protein: 22 grams

Fat: 11 grams

Mixed Spice Burgers

Difficulty Level: 2/5

Preparation & Cooking Time: 25-30 minutes

Servings: 6/2 chops each

Ingredients:

Medium onion (1)

Fresh parsley (3 tbsp.)

Clove of garlic (1)

Ground allspice (.75 tsp.)

Pepper (.75 tsp.)

Ground nutmeg (.25 tsp.)

Cinnamon (.5 tsp.)

Salt (.5 tsp.)

Fresh mint (2 tbsp.)

90% lean ground beef (1.5 lb.)

Optional: Cold Tzatziki sauce

Directions:

Finely chop/mince the parsley, mint, garlic, and onions.

Whisk the nutmeg, salt, cinnamon, pepper, allspice, garlic, mint, parsley, and onion.

Add the beef and prepare six (6) 2x4-inch oblong patties.

Use the medium temperature setting to grill the patties or broil them four inches from the heat source for four to six minutes per side.

When they're done, the meat thermometer will register 160° Fahrenheit. Serve with the sauce if desired.

Nutrition:

Calories: 231

Protein: 32 grams

Fat: 9 grams

Delicious Pork & Orzo

Difficulty Level: 2/5

Preparation & Cooking Time: 30 minutes

Servings: 6

Ingredients:

Pork tenderloin (1.5 lb.)

Olive oil (2 tbsp.)

Water (3 quarts)

Uncooked orzo pasta (1.25 cups)

Salt (.25 tsp.)

Coarsely ground pepper (1 tsp.)

Fresh baby spinach (6 oz. pkg.)

Grape tomatoes (1 cup)

Feta cheese (.75 cup)

Directions:

Rub the pork in pepper and slice the pepper into one-inch cubes.

Prepare a large skillet with oil and warm using the medium temperature setting.

Toss in the pork and cook for eight to ten minutes.

Pour water and salt in a Dutch oven and wait for it to boil. Add the orzo to simmer (lid off) for eight minutes. Stir in the spinach and cook until it's wilted and tender (45-60 sec.). Drain it in a colander.

Cut the tomatoes into halves and add in with the pork and heat, adding in the orzo mixture and crumbled feta cheese.

Nutrition:

Calories: 372

Protein: 31 grams

Fat: 11 grams

Flatbread Sandwiches

Difficulty Level: 2/5

Preparation & Cooking Time: 20 minutes

Serving Yields: 6

Ingredients Needed:

Olive oil (1 tbsp.)

7-Grain pilaf (8.5 oz. pkg.)

English seedless cucumber (1 cup)

Seeded tomato (1 cup)

Crumbled feta cheese (.25 cup)

Fresh lemon juice (2 tbsp.)

Freshly cracked black pepper (.25 tsp.)

Plain hummus (7 oz. container)

Whole grain white flatbread wraps (3 @ 2.8 oz. each)

Directions:

Cook the pilaf as directed on the package instructions and cool.

Chop and combine the tomato, cucumber, cheese, oil, pepper, and lemon juice. Fold in the pilaf.

Prepare the wraps with the hummus on one side. Spoon in the pilaf and fold.

Slice into a sandwich and serve.

Nutrition:

Calories: 310

Protein: 10 grams

Fat: 9 grams

Mezze Platter With Toasted Za'atar Pita Bread

Difficulty Level: 2/5

Preparation & Cooking Time: 10 minutes

Servings: 4

Ingredients Needed:

Whole-wheat pita rounds (4)

Olive oil (4 tbsp.)

Za'atar (4 tsp.)

Greek yogurt (1 cup)

Black pepper & Kosher salt (to your liking)

Hummus (1 cup)

Marinated artichoke hearts (1 cup)

Assorted olives (2 cups)

Sliced roasted red peppers (1 cup)

Cherry tomatoes (2 cups)

Salami (4 oz.)

Directions:

Use the medium-high heat setting to heat a large skillet.

Lightly brush the pita bread with the oil on each side and add the za'atar for seasoning.

Prepare in batches by adding the pita into a skillet and toasting until browned. It should take about two minutes on each side. Slice each of the pitas into quarters.

Season the yogurt with pepper and salt.

To assemble, divide the potatoes and add the hummus, yogurt, artichoke hearts, olives, red peppers, tomatoes, and salami.

Nutrition:

Calories: 731

Protein: 26 grams

Fat: 48 grams

Mediterranean Whole Wheat Pizza

Difficulty Level: 2/5

Preparation & Cooking Time: 25 minutes

Servings: 4

Ingredients:

Whole-wheat pizza crust (1)

Basil pesto (4 oz. jar)

Artichoke hearts (.5 cup)

Kalamata olives (2 tbsp.)

Pepperoncini (2 tbsp. drained)

Feta cheese (.25 cup)

Directions:

Program the oven to 450° Fahrenheit.

Drain and pull the artichokes to pieces. Slice/chop the pepperoncini and olives.

Arrange the pizza crust onto a floured work surface and cover it using pesto. Arrange the artichoke, pepperoncini slices, and olives over the pizza. Lastly, crumble and add the feta.

Bake in the hot oven until the cheese has melted, and it has a crispy crust or 10-12 minutes.

Nutrition:

Calories: 277

Protein: 9.7 grams

Fat: 18.6 grams

Spinach & Feta Pita Bake

Difficulty Level: 2/5

Preparation & Cooking Time: 22 minutes

Servings: 6

Ingredients:

Sun-dried tomato pesto (6 oz. tub)

Roma - plum tomatoes (2 chopped)

Whole-wheat pita bread (Six 6-inch)

Spinach (1 bunch)

Mushrooms (4 sliced)

Grated Parmesan cheese (2 tbsp.)

Crumbled feta cheese (.5 cup)

Olive oil (3 tbsp.)

Black pepper (as desired)

Directions:

Set the oven at 350° Fahrenheit.

Spread the pesto onto one side of each pita bread and arrange them onto a baking tray (pesto-side up).

Rinse and chop the spinach. Top the pitas with spinach, mushrooms, tomatoes, feta cheese, pepper, Parmesan cheese, pepper, and a drizzle of oil.

Bake in the hot oven until the pita bread is crispy (12 min.). Slice the pitas into quarters.

Nutritional Information:

- Calories: 350
- Protein: 11.6 grams
- Fat: 17.1g rams

Watermelon Feta & Balsamic Pizza

Difficulty Level: 2/5

Preparation & Cooking Time: 15 minutes

Servings: 4

Ingredients:

Watermelon (1-inch thick from the center)

Crumbled feta cheese (1 oz.)

Sliced Kalamata olives (5-6)

Mint leaves (1 tsp.)

Balsamic glaze (.5 tbsp.)

Directions:

Slice the widest section of the watermelon in half. Then, slice each half into four wedges.

Serve on a round pie dish like a pizza round and cover with the olives, cheese, mint leaves, and glaze.

Nutritional Information:

- Protein: 2 grams
- Fat: 3 grams
- Calories: 90

Lentil, Shrimp and Bean Salad

Difficulty Level: 2/5

Preparation Time: 10 minutes

Cooking Time: 5 minutes

Servings: 4

Ingredients:

.5 bell pepper, chopped

5-7 mint leaves, chopped

2 tspn capers

2 tspn garlic, minced

1 can brown lentils ~15 oz

7 oz cooked shrimp

2 tbsp white wine vinegar

1 can white beans ~15 oz

salt and black pepper to taste

2 tbsp extra virgin olive oil

.5 tspn ground cumin

.5 tspn paprika

Directions:

Mix together the shrimp, pepper, capers, white beans, lentils, mint, and minced garlic.

Season with the spices and add the white wine vinegar and olive oil as a dressing.

Stir so everything is well designed.

This is a great meal with a slice of your favorite whole wheat pita bread.

Nutrition:

347 calories per serving

8.9 grams fat

38 grams carbs

19.5 grams protein

Spinach and egg scramble with raspberries

Difficulty Level: 2/5

Preparation Time: 10 minutes

Cooking Time: 10 minutes

Servings: 1

Ingredients:

One teaspoon of canola oil

One and a half cups of baby spinach (which is one and a half ounces)

Two eggs, large and lightly beaten

Kosher salt, a pinch.

Ground pepper, a pinch

One slice of whole-grain toasted bread

Half cup of fresh and fine raspberries

Directions:

Heat the oil in a non-stick and small skillet at a temperature of medium-high.

Add spinach to the plate.

Cleanly wipe the pan and add eggs into the medium heated pan.

Stir and cook twice in order to ensure even-cooking for about two minutes.

Stir the spinach in and add salt and pepper into it.

Garnish it with raspberries and toast before eating.

Nutrition:

Carbohydrate - 21 g

Protein - 18 g

Fat - 16 g

Calories: 296 calories

Mediterranean lettuce wraps

Difficulty Level: 2/5

Preparation Time: 10 minutes

Cooking Time: 10 minutes

Servings: 4

Ingredients:

One-fourth cup of tahini

One-fourth cup of olive oil, extra-virgin

One teaspoon of lemon zest

One-fourth cup of lemon juice

One and a half tsp. of pure maple syrup

Three fourth tsp. of kosher salt

Half tsp. of paprika

Two cans (15 ounces) of rinsed chickpeas, no-salt-added

Half cup of sliced and roasted red pepper - drained and jarred

Half cup of thinly sliced shallots

Twelve leaves of Bibb lettuce, large

One-fourth cup of almonds, roasted and chopped

Two tsp. of fresh parsley, chopped

Directions:

Whisk lemon zest, tahini, oil, maple syrup, lemon juice, paprika, and all in a bowl.

After which, add peppers, chickpeas, and shallots.

Now, toss for coating.

After this, divide this mixture among the lettuce leaves (say about one-third cup for every portion).

Top with parsley and almonds.

Before serving, wrap lettuce leaves around this filling for proper garnishing.

Nutrition:

Carbohydrate - 44 g

Protein - 16 g

Fat - 28 g

Calories: 498 calories

Shrimp, Avocado and Feta Wrap

Difficulty Level: 2/5

Preparation Time: 5 minutes

Cooking Time: 5 minutes

Servings: 2

Ingredients:

Chopped cooked shrimp (3 ounces)

Lime juice (1 tablespoon)

Crumbled feta cheese (2 tablespoons)

Diced avocado (¼ cup)

Whole-wheat tortilla (1 piece)

Diced tomato (¼ cup)

Sliced scallion (1 Piece)

Directions:

Spray vegetable oil on a skillet and then heat it. Add the shrimp to get a nice pink color to them.

Add the feta cheese on one side of the wrap and also be generous with the cheese.

Top the cheese with the various other ingredients. Add the shrimp on the top so they will be in the middle of the wrap when you roll it.

Add lime juice to give it the tangy zing to the wrap.

Then roll the wrap tightly, but make sure that the ingredients don't fall off.

Then cut the wrap in two halves and serve it.

Nutrition:

Carbohydrate – 34 g

Protein - 29 g

Fat – 14 g

Calories: 371

Greek Salad Nachos

Difficulty Level: 2/5

Preparation Time: 15 minutes

Cooking Time: 15 minutes

Servings: 6

Ingredients:

A ⅓ cup of hummus

2 tablespoons of extra-virgin olive oil

1 tablespoon of lemon juice

¼ teaspoon of ground pepper

3 cups of whole-grain pita chips

1 cup of chopped lettuce

A ½ cup of quartered grape tomatoes

A ¼ cup of crumbled feta cheese

2 tablespoons of chopped olives

2 tablespoons of minced red onion

1 tablespoon of minced fresh oregano

Directions:

Whisk pepper, lemon juice, oil, and hummus in a bowl.

Spread the pita chips on a plate in one layer.

Cover the chips with about ¾ of that hummus mix and top it with tomatoes, red onion, olives, feta, and lettuce. Cover it with the rest of the hummus. Sprinkle oregano on top before serving it.

Nutrition:

Carbohydrate – 13 g

Protein – 4 g

Fat – 10 g

Calories: 159 calories

Sirloin with Sweet Bell Peppers

Difficulty Level: 2/5

Preparation Time: 20 minutes

Cooking Time: 8 minutes

Servings: 4

Ingredients:

12 ounces boneless top sirloin steak, about 1-inch thick, trimmed of visible fat

1 tablespoon olive oil, divided

Sea salt

Freshly ground black pepper

1 yellow bell pepper, thinly sliced

1 red bell pepper, thinly sliced

1 orange bell pepper, thinly sliced

1 small red onion, thinly sliced

4 garlic cloves, crushed

Juice of 1 lemon

Directions:

Preheat the oven to broil.

Lightly oil the steak on both sides with 1 teaspoon of olive oil and season with salt and pepper. Place the steak on a baking sheet.

In a large bowl, toss together the bell peppers, onion, garlic, and remaining 2 teaspoons of olive oil. Season lightly with salt and pepper. Spread the vegetables on the baking sheet around the steak.

Broil the steak and vegetables until the steak is browned and the desired doneness, turning once, about 4 minutes per side.

Remove from the oven and let the steak rest for 10 minutes. Slice thinly on the bias against the grain. Drizzle the vegetables with lemon juice and serve.

Nutrition:

Calories: 170

Total fat: 7g

Saturated fat: 2g

Carbohydrates: 11g

Sugar: 2g

Fiber: 2g

Protein: 18g

Quinoa and Spinach Salad with Figs and Balsamic Dressing

Difficulty Level: 2/5

Preparation Time: 10 minutes, plus cooling time

Cooking Time: *15 minutes*

Servings: 4

Ingredients:

½ cup quinoa

1 cup water

6 cups chopped spinach

8 ripe figs, quartered

¼ cup sunflower seeds

½ cup store-bought balsamic dressing

½ cup crumbled goat cheese

Directions:

Rinse the quinoa under cold running water to remove its bitter flavor. In a small saucepan, combine the quinoa and water and bring to a boil over medium heat. Reduce the heat to low and simmer, uncovered, until the liquid is absorbed, 10 to 15 minutes. Transfer to a dish and refrigerate until cool.

In a large bowl, toss the spinach, cooled quinoa, figs, and sunflower seeds until well mixed. Add the dressing, toss to coat, and transfer the salad to serving plates. Top with goat cheese and serve.

Nutrition:

Calories: 348

Total fat: 12g

Saturated fat: 3g

Carbohydrates: 54g

Sugar: 21g

Fiber: 7g

Protein: 11g

Greek-Style Tuna Salad in Pita

Difficulty Level: 2/5

Preparation Time: *25 minutes*

Cooking Time: *0 minutes*

Servings: *4*

Ingredients:

2 (5-ounce) cans water-packed tuna, drained

½ English cucumber, chopped

1 yellow bell pepper, chopped

¼ cup chopped oil-packed sun-dried tomatoes

2 tablespoons pitted, chopped Kalamata olives

2 tablespoons chopped fresh parsley

1 tablespoon freshly squeezed lemon juice

Sea salt

Freshly ground black pepper

4 whole-wheat pita bread rounds, halved

½ cup crumbled feta cheese

1 cup shredded Boston lettuce

Directions:

In a large bowl, stir together the tuna, cucumber, bell pepper, sun-dried tomatoes, olives, parsley, and lemon juice. Season with salt and pepper.

Scoop the tuna salad into the pita halves and top them with feta cheese and lettuce. Serve.

Nutrition:

Calories: 192

Total fat: 6g

Saturated fat: 3g

Carbohydrates: 23g

Sugar: 5g

Fiber: 3g

Protein: 14g

Delicious Broccoli Tortellini Salad

Difficulty Level: 2/5

Preparation Time: *10 minutes*

Cooking Time: *20 to 25 minutes*

Servings: *12*

Ingredients:

1 cup sunflower seeds, or any of your favorite seeds

3 heads of broccoli, fresh is best!

½ cup sugar

20 ounces cheese-filled tortellini

1 onion

2 teaspoons cider vinegar

½ cup mayonnaise

1 cup raisins-optional

Directions:

Cut your broccoli into florets and chop the onion.

Follow the directions to make the cheese-filled tortellini. Once they are cooked, drain and rinse them with cold water.

In a bowl, combine your mayonnaise, sugar, and vinegar. Whisk well to give the ingredients a dressing consistency.

In a separate large bowl, toss in your seeds, onion, tortellini, raisins, and broccoli.

Pour the salad dressing into the large bowl and toss the ingredients together. You will want to ensure everything is thoroughly mixed as you'll want a taste of the salad dressing with every bite!

Nutrition:

Calories: 272

Fats: 8.1 Grams

Carbohydrates: 38.6 Grams

Protein: 5 Grams

Tuna and Cheese Bake

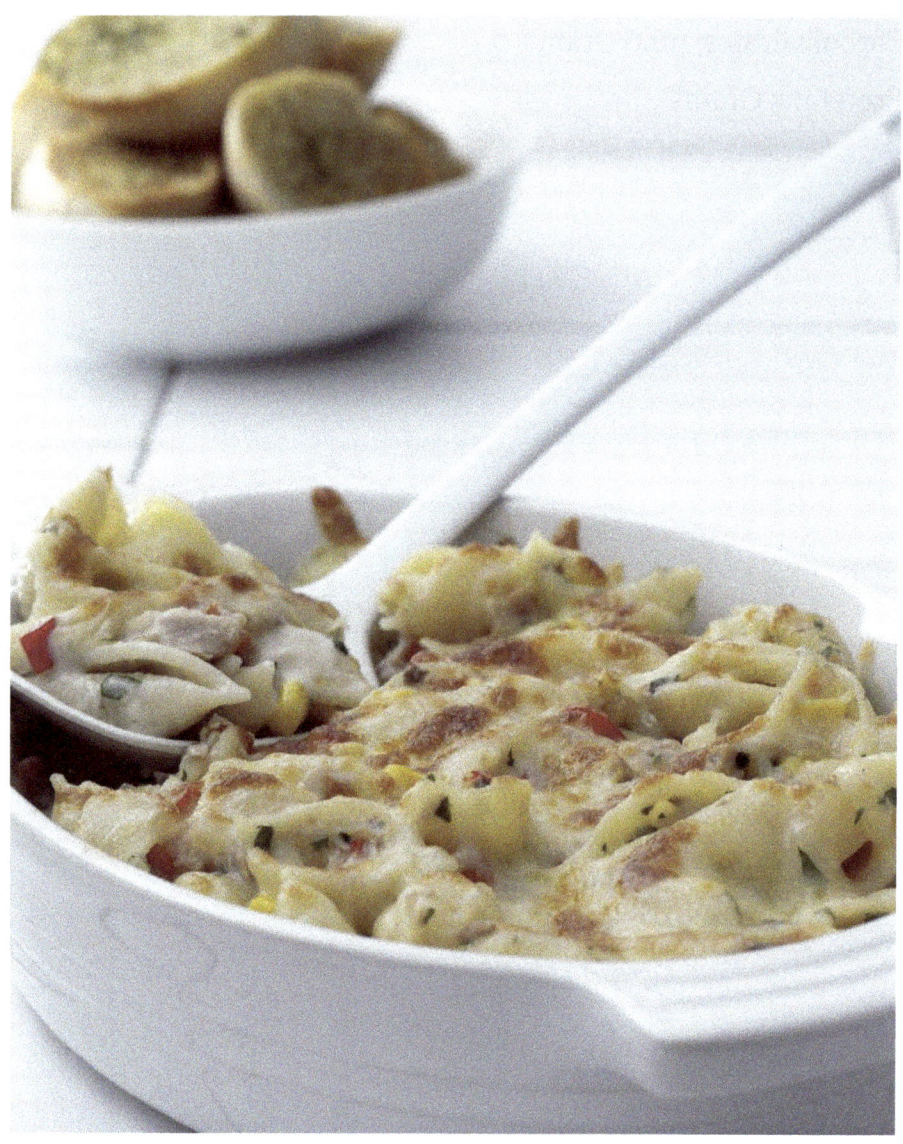

Difficulty Level: 2/5

Preparation time: *5 minutes*

Cooking time: *15 minutes*

Servings: 4

Ingredients:

10 ounces canned tuna, drained and flaked

4 eggs, whisked

½ cup feta cheese, shredded

1 tablespoon chives, chopped

1 tablespoon parsley, chopped

Salt and black pepper to the taste

3 teaspoons olive oil

Directions:

Grease a baking dish with the oil, add the tuna and the rest of the ingredients except the cheese, toss and bake at 370 degrees F for 15 minutes.

Sprinkle the cheese on top, leave the mix aside for 5 minutes, slice and serve for breakfast.

Nutrition:

Calories 283

Fat 14.2

Fiber 5.6

Carbs 12.1

Protein 6.4

Pressure Pot Potato Salad

Difficulty Level: 2/5

Preparation time: *5 minutes,*

Cook Time: 10 minutes

Servings: 2

Ingredients:

6 potatoes, peeled and cubed

4 eggs

1 cup mayonnaise

1 tablespoon dill pickle juice

Salt and pepper for taste

2 cups water

¼ cup chopped onion

2 tablespoons chopped parsley

1 tablespoon muster

Directions:

Take your steamer basket and put it in pressure cooker pot.

Add the water, potatoes, and eggs, and then cook on high pressure for 4 minutes.

When finished, pull the eggs out and let them cool in cold water.

Add the other ingredients together, and then the cooled potatoes and mix it in. you can then dice the eggs and put it in the salad, and then add salt and pepper for taste. Let it chill for an hour if you want that.

Nutrition:

Calories: 230,

Fat: 9 g

Carbs: 22g

Net Carbs: 15 g

Protein: 12 g

Fiber: 7 g.

Sodium 117mg

Veggie Hummus Sandwich

Difficulty Level: 2/5

Preparation Time: *10 minutes*

Cooking Time: *10 minutes*

Servings: *2*

Ingredients:

4 slices of whole-grain bread

6 tbsp of hummus

1 cup of salad greens or spinach

½ cup of shredded carrot

½ medium bell pepper halved

½ cup of cucumber, sliced

½ avocado, mashed

Directions:

Combine all the ingredients together in a small mixing bowl. Spread hummus over a piece of toast or pita bread. Pour the mixture of cucumber, carrot, bell pepper, and greens in the sandwich. Then, cut the sandwich in half or quarters and serve or put in a plastic bag ready for your lunch at work or school.

Nutrition:

Calories: 320

Fat: 14g

Carbs: 40g

Spicy Potato Salad

Difficulty Level: 2/5

Preparation time: *10 minutes*

Cooking time: *15 minutes*

Servings: 4

Ingredients:

1 and ½ pounds baby potatoes, peeled and halved

A pinch of salt and black pepper

2 tablespoons harissa paste

6 ounces Greek yogurt

Juice of 1 lemon

¼ cup red onion, chopped

¼ cup parsley, chopped

Directions:

Put the potatoes in a pot, add water to cover, add salt, bring to a boil over medium-high heat, cook for 12 minutes, drain and transfer them to a bowl.

Add the harissa and the rest of the ingredients, toss and serve for lunch.

Nutrition:

Calories 354

Fat 19.2

Fiber 4.5

Carbs 24.7

Protein 11.2

Tomato and Halloumi Platter

Difficulty Level: 2/5

Preparation time: *5 minutes*

Cooking time: *4 minutes*

Servings: 4

Ingredients:

1-pound tomatoes, sliced

½ pound halloumi, cut into 4 slices

2 tablespoons parsley, chopped

1 tablespoon basil, chopped

2 tablespoons olive oil

A pinch of salt and black pepper

Juice of 1 lemon

Directions:

Brush the halloumi slices with half of the oil, put them on your preheated grill and cook over medium-high heat and cook for 2 minutes on each side.

Arrange the tomato slices on a platter, season with salt and pepper, drizzle the lemon juice and the rest of the oil all over, top with the halloumi slices, sprinkle the herbs on top and serve for lunch.

Nutrition:

Calories 181

Fat 7.3

Fiber 1.4

Carbs 4.6

Protein 1.1

Bean Lettuce Wraps

Difficulty Level: 2/5

Preparation Time: *5 minutes*

Cooking Time: *20 minutes*

Servings: *4*

Ingredients:

8 Romaine lettuce leaves

½ cup Garlic hummus or any prepared hummus

¾ cup chopped tomatoes

15 ounce can great northern beans, drained and rinsed

½ cup diced onion

1 tablespoon extra-virgin olive oil

¼ cup chopped parsley

¼ teaspoon black pepper

Directions:

Set a skillet on top of the stove range over medium heat.

In the skillet, warm the oil for a couple of minutes.

Add the onion into the oil. Stir frequently as the onion cooks for a few minutes.

Combine the pepper and tomatoes and cook for another couple of minutes. Remember to stir occasionally.

Add the beans and continue to stir and cook for 2 to 3 minutes.

Turn the burner off, remove the skillet from heat, and add the parsley.

Set the lettuce leaves on a flat surface and spread 1 tablespoon of hummus on each leaf.

Divide the bean mixture onto the 8 leaves.

Spread the bean mixture down the center of the leaves.

Fold the leaves by starting lengthwise on one side.

Fold over the other side so the leaf is completely wrapped.

Serve and enjoy!

Nutrition:

Calories: 211

Fats: 8 Grams

Carbohydrates: 28 Grams

Protein: 10 Grams

Margherita Mediterranean Model

Difficulty Level: 2/5

Preparation time: 15 minutes

Cooking time: 15 minutes

Servings: 10

Ingredients:

1-batch pizza shell

2-tbsp olive oil

½-cup crushed tomatoes

3-Roma tomatoes, sliced ¼-inch thick

½-cup fresh basil leaves, thinly sliced

6-oz. block mozzarella, cut into ¼-inch slices, blot-dry with a paper towel

½-tsp sea salt

Directions:

Preheat your oven to 450 °F.

Lightly brush the pizza shell with olive oil. Thoroughly spread the crushed tomatoes over the pizza shell, leaving a half-inch space around its edge as the crust.

Top the pizza with the Roma tomato slices, basil leaves, and mozzarella slices. Sprinkle salt over the pizza.

Place the pizza directly on the oven rack. Bake for 15 minutes until the cheese is bubbling and melting from the center to the edge. Let the pizza cool for 5 minutes before slicing.

Nutrition:

Calories: 251

Total Fats: 8g

Fiber: 1g

Carbohydrates: 34g

Protein: 9g

Very Vegan Patras Pasta

Difficulty Level: 2/5

Preparation time: 5 minutes

Cooking time: 10 minutes

Servings: 6

Ingredients:

4-quarts salted water

10-oz. gluten-free and whole grain pasta

5-cloves garlic, minced

1-cup hummus

Salt and pepper

⅓-cup water

½-cup walnuts

½-cup olives

2-tbsp dried cranberries (optional)

Directions:

Bring the salted water to a boil for cooking the pasta.

In the meantime, prepare for the hummus sauce. Combine the garlic, hummus, salt, and pepper with water in a mixing bowl. Add the walnuts, olive, and dried cranberries, if desired. Set aside.

Add the pasta in the boiling water. Cook the pasta in accordance with the manufacturer's specifications until attaining an *al dente* texture. Drain the pasta.

Transfer the pasta to a large serving bowl and combine with the sauce.

Nutrition:

Calories: 329

Total Fats: 12.6g

Fiber: 7.9g

Carbohydrates: 43.3g

Protein: 12g

Tangy Tilapia Fish Fillets with Crusty Coating

Difficulty Level: 2/5

Preparation time: 5 minutes

Cooking time: 10 minutes

Servings: 4

Ingredients:

¼-cup ground flaxseed

1-cup almonds, finely chopped (divided)

4-6 oz. tilapia fillets

½-tsp salt

2-tbsp olive oil

Directions:

Combine the flaxseed with half of the almonds in a shallow mixing bowl to serve as a crusty coating, instead of a flour mixture.

Sprinkle the tilapia fillets evenly with salt. Dredge the fillet in the flaxseed-almond mixture. Set aside.

Heat the olive oil in a heavy, thick-bottomed skillet placed over medium heat. Add the coated fillets, and cook for 4 minutes on each side until golden brown, flipping once. Remove the fillets, and transfer them in a serving plate.

In the same skillet, add the remaining almonds. Toast for a minute until turning golden brown, stirring frequently.

To serve, sprinkle the toasted almonds over the fish fillets.

Nutrition:

Calories: 258

Total Fats: 21.3g

Fiber: 4.9g

Carbohydrates: 7.1g

Protein: 11.6g

Feta-Fused Mussels Marmite

Difficulty Level: 2/5

Preparation time: 10 minutes

Cooking time: 20 minutes

Servings: 6

Ingredients:

2-tbsp olive oil

1-pc medium onion, chopped

1-cup white wine

½-tsp salt

2-lbs mussels (without the shell)

1-dash of cayenne pepper

2-cloves of garlic, chopped

1-tbsp tomato paste

2-oz of feta cheese grated

Bunch of parsley, chopped

Directions:

Preheat your oven to 400 °F.

Heat the oil in a large pot placed over medium-high heat and sauté the onion for 3 minutes until tender. Pour the white wine, and add the tomato, salt, and mussels. Bring to a boil until all the mussels break open and the wine evaporates.

Add the cayenne and garlic. Simmer for 5 minutes.

Take out the top shell of the mussels. Sprinkle the opened mussels with feta cheese and parsley.

Place the pot in the preheated oven. Grill for 8 minutes until the cheese begins to melt and appear with a golden color.

TIP: Remove any closed mussel; a closed one is an indication that it is bad!

Nutrition:

Calories: 227

Total Fats: 10.1g

Fiber: 0.6g

Carbohydrates: 9.8g

Protein: 19.8g

Sauced Shellfish in White Wine

Difficulty Level: 3/5

Preparation time: 10 minutes

Cooking time: 10 minutes

Servings: 6

Ingredients:

2-lbs fresh cuttlefish

½-cup olive oil

1-pc large onion, finely chopped

1-cup of Robola white wine

¼-cup lukewarm water

1-pc bay leaf

½-bunch parsley, chopped

4-pcs tomatoes, grated

Salt and pepper

Directions:

Take out the hard centerpiece of cartilage (cuttlebone), the bag of ink, and the intestines from the cuttlefish. Wash the cleaned cuttlefish with running water. Slice it into small pieces, and drain excess water.

Heat the oil in a saucepan placed over medium-high heat and sauté the onion for 3 minutes until tender. Add the sliced cuttlefish and pour in the white wine. Cook for 5 minutes until it simmers.

Pour in the water, and add the tomatoes, bay leaf, parsley, tomatoes, salt, and pepper. Simmer the mixture over low heat until the cuttlefish slices are tender and left with their thick sauce. Serve them warm with rice.

TIP: Be careful not to overcook the cuttlefish as its texture becomes very hard. A safe rule of thumb is grilling the cuttlefish over a ragingly hot fire for 3 minutes before using it in any recipe.

Nutrition:

Calories: 308

Total Fats: 18.1g

Fiber: 1.5g

Carbohydrates: 8g

Protein: 25.6g

Minty Melon & Fruity Feta with Cool Cucumber

Difficulty Level: 1/5

Preparation time: 15 minutes

Cooking time: 0 minutes

Servings: 4

Ingredients:

3-cups watermelon cubes

2-pcs tomatoes, diced

1-pc lemon, zested and juiced

1-pc cucumber, peeled, seeded & diced

½-cup fresh mint, roughly chopped

½-bulb red onion, sliced

¼-cup olive oil

Salt and pepper

⅓-cup crumbled feta cheese

Directions:

Combine and mix the watermelon, tomatoes, lemon juice, lemon zest, cucumber, mint, red onion, and olive oil in a large mixing bowl. Sprinkle over the salt and pepper. Toss to combine evenly.

Serve chilled with a sprinkling of crumbled feta cheese.

Nutrition:

Calories: 205

Total Fats: 15.5g

Fiber: 3.3g

Carbohydrates: 18.5g

Protein: 3.7g

Limassolian Lemony Steamed Spears with Cheese Chips

Difficulty Level: 2/5

Preparation time: 2 minutes

Cooking time: 6 minutes

Servings: 4

Ingredients:

1-bunch asparagus

1-tbsp olive oil

Salt and pepper

2-pcs fresh lemons

2-tbsp Mediterranean herb feta crumbled cheese

Directions:

Place the asparagus spears in your steamer. Cover the steamer, and steam for 6 minutes until tender.

Arrange the steamed spears on a serving platter. Toss with olive oil, salt, and freshly squeezed lemons.

To serve, garnish with lemon wedges and sprinkle with feta cheese.

Nutrition:

Calories: 45

Total Fats: 1g

Fiber: 5g

Carbohydrates: 11g

Protein: 3g

Oven-grilled Oyster Mushroom Meal

Difficulty Level: 2/5

Preparation time: 10 minutes

Cooking time: 15 minutes

Servings: 4

Ingredients:

20-oz. oyster mushrooms

2-tbsp extra-virgin olive oil

Salt and freshly ground pepper

2-tsp parsley, minced

Directions:

Preheat your oven to 420 °F.

Line a 5" x 9" baking sheet with foil, and spray the surfaces with non-stick grease. Set aside.

Meanwhile, prepare the mushrooms by separating and discarding their stems. By using a damp towel or a mushroom brush, clean their top surfaces.

Spray or brush the mushrooms with the olive oil. Place and arrange the mushrooms in a baking sheet. Grill for 5 minutes. (Grill for an additional 4 minutes for thicker mushrooms.

Take out the sheet, and place the grilled mushrooms in a serving platter. Sprinkle over with salt and freshly ground pepper. Top them with parsley, and serve immediately.

Nutrition:

Calories: 107

Total Fats: 7.3g

Fiber: 3.3g

Carbohydrates: 8.7g

Protein: 4.7g

Grilled Burgers with Mushrooms

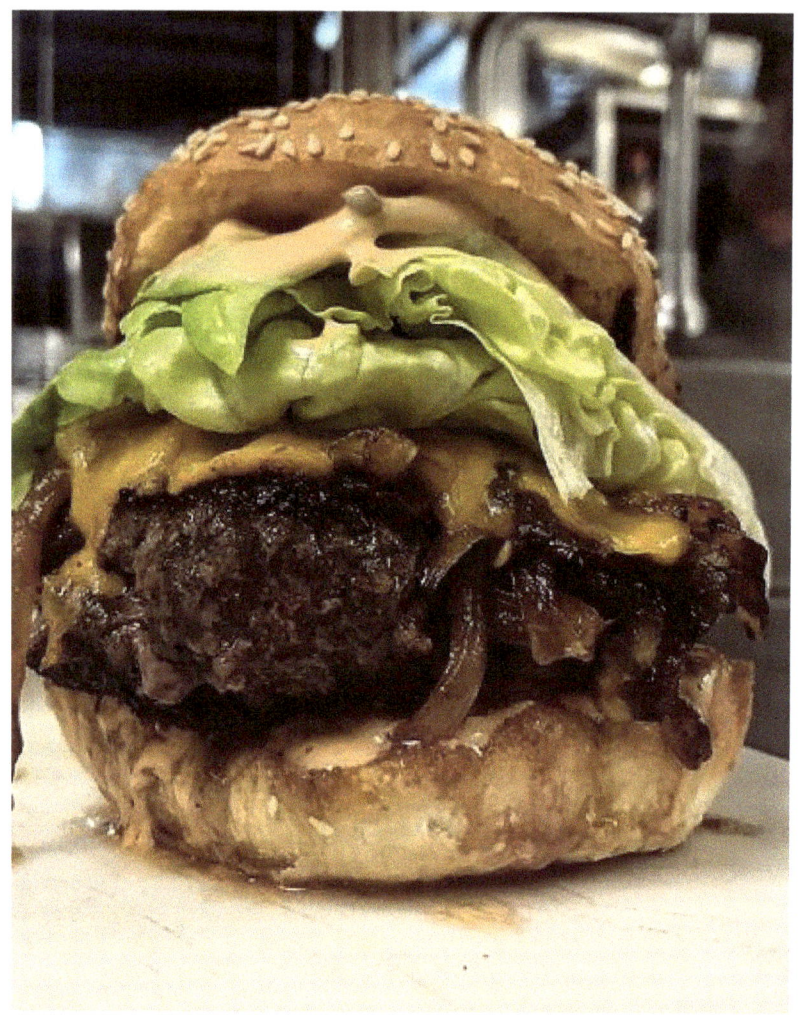

Difficulty Level: 2/5

Preparation time: 10 minutes

Cooking time: 10 minutes

Servings: 4

Ingredients:

2 Bibb lettuce, halved

4 slices red onion

4 slices tomato

4 whole wheat buns, toasted

2 tbsp olive oil

¼ tsp cayenne pepper, optional

1 garlic clove, minced

1 tbsp sugar

½ cup water

1/3 cup balsamic vinegar

4 large Portobello mushroom caps, around 5-inches in diameter

Directions:

Remove stems from mushrooms and clean with a damp cloth. Transfer into a baking dish with gill-side up.

In a bowl, mix thoroughly olive oil, cayenne pepper, garlic, sugar, water and vinegar. Pour over mushrooms and marinate mushrooms in the ref for at least an hour.

Once the one hour is nearly up, preheat grill to medium high fire and grease grill grate.

Grill mushrooms for five minutes per side or until tender. Baste mushrooms with marinade so it doesn't dry up.

To assemble, place ½ of bread bun on a plate, top with a slice of onion, mushroom, tomato and one lettuce leaf. Cover with the other top half of the bun. Repeat process with remaining ingredients, serve and enjoy.

Nutrition:

Calories: 244.1

Fiber: 9.3g

Carbohydrates: 32g

Protein: 8.1g

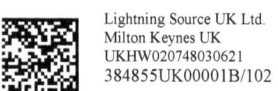

Lightning Source UK Ltd.
Milton Keynes UK
UKHW020748030621
384855UK00001B/102